COMPARIN

IMMU

VACCINATION

by Trevor Gunn

CONTENTS

COMPARING NATURAL
IMMUNITY WITH VACCINATION

Questioning an established practice such as vaccination may on the surface seem like a vast and complicated task. However if we start by asking some of the basic questions, such as, what is the rationale of vaccinating, why and how was this method popularised, are germs really the source of disease, and what role has vaccination played in the fall of infectious diseases, then this complex subject begins to unfold into a much simpler issue.

A BRIEF HISTORY

If we look back to the nineteenth century we can observe how much of our current medical ideas were developing - the time when scientific thinking began to dominate over many accepted religious beliefs, such as, how did life begin and how did we get here?

Two scientists in 19th century France, Louis Pasteur and Antoine Bechamp, were particularly interested in trying to understand disease processes, and two main schools of thought began to emerge. Pasteur held a 'creationist' view - spontaneous generation - believing that life and disease processes could happen from nothing. Whereas Bechamp held an 'evolutionist' view - meaning that all disease processes evolved from what was already there. Through his research Bechamp discovered 'microzymas' that were involved in disease processes (some of which we now know as micro-organisms) and that these particles were already present within the body and that there need not be an infection from outside of the body to cause disease. It was these micro-organisms that could initiate fermentation, decay and disease by virtue of their metabolism in a suitable environment.

Pasteur is often wrongly credited with having discovered that micro-organisms cause disease and can be transferred from person to person by the passage of micro-organisms through the air. The action of the microbe was however discovered by Bechamp and although micro-organisms, bacteria, fungus etc can be transferred through the air, Bechamp made it very clear that the micro-organisms that are associated with illness do not cause the illness but merely accumulate if the conditions in the individual support those particular micro-organisms. Basically, micro-organisms live off a toxic internal milieu and can actually help to clean up the environment.

Pasteur, on seeing Bechamp's results, formulated the idea that for each particular process there must be a separate kind of micro-organism responsible for the disease, this gave birth to his *Germ Theory of Disease;* again, a doctrine that had been formulated long before Pasteur had claimed it to be his own. According to 'germ theory' specific micro-organisms would cause specific diseases by entering the body from an external source, hence the term 'infection'; coming from outside to in.

These two interpretations of illness lead to two very different views of the cause, treatment, and prevention of disease. If we are to accept Pasteur's theory, believing that the infecting germ is the most important part of the equation, what do we have to do with regards to treating illness?

We have to kill or protect ourselves from the germ. Consequently the germ becomes synonymous with the disease; we talk about the germ and the disease as if they were the same thing. We must kill the germ or avoid contamination (i.e. avoid contact with anyone that has the germ), because the supposition is that the germ is the cause.

Alternatively, what are the consequences of accepting Bechamp's theory, that the micro-organisms are already present and that it is the state of health, the internal environment, which will affect the proliferation of bacteria and virus?

Then we must improve the internal environment- the 'soil'. In terms of the human condition we need to look specifically at toxicity, diet, lifestyle, emotional state and mental stress. If you change the 'soil', you will change the nature of the environment that the germs live in, consequently you will change the type of germs present and you will also change the nature of the waste products that these germs generate, i.e. changing the soil will also change the toxins that the germs produce.

So what medical paradigm did we adopt, who did we choose to invest in? It was of course Pasteur, yes there were many social improvements that came, but they came as a result of social reform not medical insight, our medical philosophy has stayed squarely within the doctrine of Pasteur.

WHY HAVE WE SO HEAVILY INVESTED IN THIS MEDICAL PARADIGM?

There may be several reasons for this, one of which was not the actual efficacy of the approach; there were many examples of communities and individuals adopting the Bechamp approach that were in fact more successful than Pasteur. However, it appears easier to blame a germ as being the cause of your condition and therefore easier to embrace the views of Pasteur, rather than acknowledging the real causes of disease, i.e. poor diet, toxins and lifestyle. In the Pasteur paradigm, you need not take any responsibility for your health and ill-health, so psychologically it was easier to make Pasteur right - we wanted him to be right.

Socially and economically during the 19th century and the time of the Industrial revolution, it was standard medical text to acknowledge that the appalling living conditions were the causes of illnesses prevalent at that time. However, factory owners and land owners, the wealthy friends of government were far too interested in profit to address the living and working conditions of the new working class, economically and politically the medical paradigm of Pasteur received much greater support than that of Bechamp.

Now let's turn briefly to Edward Jenner, the so-called father of vaccination. He apparently observed that milkmaids who had cowpox (a skin affection from the udders of cows), would very rarely get smallpox, it was therefore presumed that the immune response to cowpox was similar to the immune response to smallpox. It was then further deduced that if you were immune to one you would be immune to both. Edward Jenner therefore tried to create an extraction of cowpox, later termed a vaccination (vaccinia = Latin : cow) and inject this into individuals in the hope of stimulating an immune response to cowpox that would subsequently also work against smallpox.

Cowpox was seen as a milder disease than smallpox and inoculation with cowpox was seen as a way of gaining immunity to the more 'dangerous' smallpox. In 1796 Jenner promoted that idea and the use of a vaccine, and the more popular history books credit Edward Jenner with the invention of vaccination, this procedure was however in existence throughout Europe at least 140 years before and in other parts of the world before that.

So from Pasteur we are saying that disease is caused by something that comes from the outside and gets into our body, and with Jenner we are saying that some of those germs are more dangerous than others. Each time we are handing more power to the germ, the severity of the illness is now nothing to

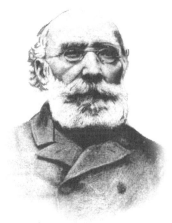

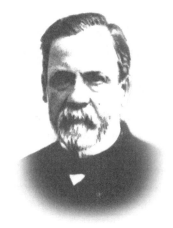

Antoine
BECHAMP
(1816-1908)

Louis
PASTEUR
(1822-1895)

EVOLUTIONIST VIEW
'Microzymas' in all living things able to evolve into bacterial forms depending on the terrain (soil)

CREATIONIST VIEW
*'Spontaneous generation'
Microbes come from the outside - invading the body*

Microbes are changeable due to environment. Pleomorphism

Microbes are non-changeable Monomorphism

THE TERRAIN THEORY
Toxicity of the 'soil' causes dis-ease

THE GERM THEORY
Microbes cause disease

ACTION NEEDED:
Change the 'soil' - address your living habits, in particular diet, living conditions, physical and emotional balance

ACTION NEEDED:
Kill the germ and/or avoid contamination, protect from the germ

do with us but to do with the power of the germ.

A quick role call of serious infectious illnesses may lead us to, polio, AIDS, meningitis, etc and of the less severe, the common cold, chicken pox, mumps, even athlete's foot. However a closer look will reveal that all of the so-called serious illnesses are associated with micro-organisms that many healthy people have within their bodies and they produce no symptoms at all - yes HIV, polio viruses, and the many micro-organisms associated with meningitis, (Hib, meningococcal, E.Coli etc) do not cause any symptoms in most people. In fact it is only in very few individuals that we even see symptoms. With the so-called less severe illnesses... well, you can die from all of them, even fungal infections that can create mild symptoms in most, can, and actually do kill others.

So although the medical paradigm - our 'germ consciousness' tells us that germs come and get us to cause disease and that some are dangerous and some are not; the reality is, any can be dangerous and all may not - clearly there is an issue of individual susceptibility that is totally missing from the germ theory.

CREATING VACCINES

Edward Jenner tried to create a vaccine for smallpox from the pustule extraction of skin eruptions in cases of cowpox. However in modern day vaccines we do not use a so-called similar disease-causing germ to produce a vaccine but we use the actual germ which is thought to be responsible for a particular disease. This is produced to make a vaccine mixture and is injected (apart from the very few oral vaccines) into the individual in the hope that they produce blood antibodies that are capable of recognizing the real pathogen should they come in contact with that pathogen later in life.

However in producing the vaccine, the pathogen i.e. the germ or toxin that we place in the vaccine mixture, must be changed slightly, so as to avoid giving the person the actual illness. Thus when injected into the individual, the immune response (the production of antibodies) would be similar enough to a response necessary to deal with the real thing, i.e. in a real disease situation. However, if the pathogen is altered too much, in the production of the vaccine, then the antibodies produced when the vaccine is administered will be made in response to something that is too different to the original, and these antibodies would not recognise the 'real' disease pathogen should it come along. This is therefore one of the inherent problems in creating vaccines; change the microbe too much and the immune response does not work against the real agent of disease, don't change enough and the vaccine itself becomes very dangerous.

Vaccines can be live, killed, acellular and genetically engineered, but whatever the procedure the primary aim would be to stimulate the production of blood antibodies for a specific disease-causing agent (pathogen), which will remain in the body to recognise and protect from future contact with these pathogens.

VACCINE SAFETY

Many of the initial vaccine safety trials were in fact only looking for symptoms of the specific disease that the vaccine would be supposedly protecting against. For instance, if a measles vaccine was produced, when looking for side-effects of the vaccine, symptoms of measles were looked for. If a measles-kind of rash appeared in individuals it was presupposed that the vaccine would require further weakening and further investigation into the side-effects of this measles vaccine would be centered on looking-out for the symptoms associated with measles.

However, since then, we have discovered that vaccines can cause all kinds of symptoms, most of which were not being looked for with the initial trials; therefore it is only more recently that we are realizing the serious consequences of vaccines. Although vaccinators are using what they believe to be the cause of measles when they create the vaccine, the process of vaccinating, by injecting pathogens into the body is not the manner in which the disease is contracted naturally, it is actually more similar to a poisonous bite than measles, consequently the symptoms associated with the adverse effects of the vaccine are different than the disease you are vaccinating against.

The other problem with regards to safety is that there are strict time limits for the period in which reactions can be attributed to the vaccine. For example, with live vaccines you are allowed fourteen days to react, killed vaccines you only have 72 hours in which to react. If you react outside of these time periods then the adverse effects will not be acknowledged as being caused by the vaccine. So this narrows the criteria in which we see adverse events, as many reactions may fall out of these time limits, some taking many weeks, months and years to fully manifest.

EFFECTIVENESS

As for trials relating to the effectiveness of a vaccine, we need to be aware that the phase one trials that often publicise the effectiveness of vaccines tend to be test-tube studies, mainly concerning antibodies; these are often quoted as efficacy rates of the vaccine. However these trials are inadequate, as they do not actually tell you what would happen in a real disease situation. Even if antibodies produced by the vaccine recipient do help in a real disease, there is a big assumption that they alone will protect the individual. The immune system is far more complex, and even now, still incompletely understood. For example it is possible to have high levels of antibody and not be immune. Equally it is possible to have no detectable levels of antibody and not get the disease. Do you think the medical profession would agree with that?

The question as regards to antibodies and immunity was posed to Dr John Clements leader of the WHO EPI (World Health Organisation, Expanded Program on Immunisation) in a letter of September 1995.

Dr Clements agrees and it is recognised that an individual may have no or almost immeasurable levels of antibodies and be immune and similarly may have high levels and not be immune. Even back in 1950, a study of diphtheria conducted by the Medical Research Council in two areas of Gt. Britain found that despite having high levels of circulating antibodies some individuals contracted diphtheria, whilst others with very low levels did not.

In other words the presence of antibody is not an indication of immunity. So you cannot test anyone to see if they are immune if you are simply measuring antibody levels. Antibody levels do not indicate immunity, and they are only a small part of your blood immune response, in fact with HIV, the presence of antibody is seen as the immune system's last resort, an indication of bad prognosis and a high risk of developing symptoms of AIDS.

UK health authority spokespeople often quote the measles vaccine as being 90% effective, this actually means that 90% of the recipients will produce the so-called 'necessary' antibody levels, 90% is not a measure of vaccine effectiveness in a real disease situation, therefore it is not a statement of how effective the vaccine is at preventing disease. Similarly the necessary level of antibody is a fantasy, since there is no definition of immunity that can be defined from a certain level of antibodies. This is especially important when considering that tests for immunity to rubella involve testing for blood antibodies, which are often carried out to indicate whether the individual needs the rubella vaccine or not. However the presence of antibodies to rubella virus would be indicative of you being exposed to the virus but that does not say whether you are immune or not. That does not tell you that if you became susceptible again that you would not get rubella. This is an important point to remember, especially if discussing this issue with your GP or health visitor.

VACCINE EFFECTIVENESS - DECLINES IN DISEASE

So if we can't tell from antibodies, how do we know that vaccines have worked? We are told that vaccines have eradicated disease, or have reduced the incidence of disease or reduced the severity of disease. That smallpox vaccine wiped out smallpox, and that polio is soon to be eliminated world-wide. The Department of Health book 'Immunisation against Infectious Disease' (1990/96 editions) illustrates the effectiveness of vaccines by showing the decline in incidence of disease after the introduction of the vaccines. For example:

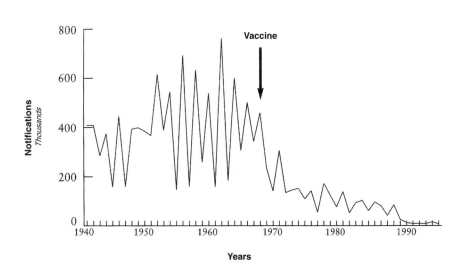

Notifications of Measles to ONS
England and Wales (1940-1995)

However to draw any worth while conclusions we need to see a 'before' and 'after', however, as many of these illnesses were not notifiable diseases the health authorities say that they do not have reliable incidence figures before 1950. Therefore we shall look at severity of illness as determined by mortality rates, the numbers of people dying of a particular illness being a good reflection of the severity of that illness. Although this is a separate statistic, the reality is that incidence and severity statistics follow parallel trends. The following graph shows the rate of decline in mortality before the introduction of the measles vaccine.

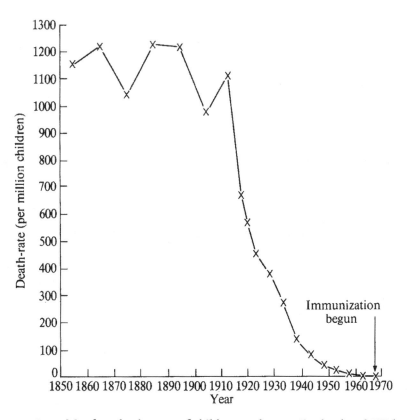

FIGURE 8.14. Measles: death rates of children under 15: England and Wales.

15

Looking at diphtheria, whooping cough, tetanus and tuberculosis. We can compare the graphs published by the U.K health authority with the OPCS they do not publish.

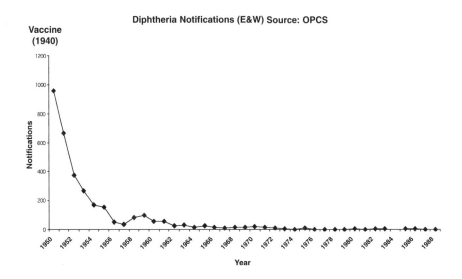

Diphtheria Notifications (E&W) Source: OPCS

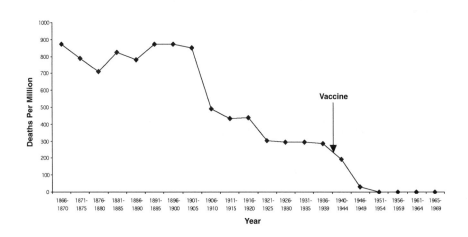

Diphtheria Deaths Per Million Children (Under 15 Years Old)

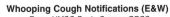

Whooping Cough Notifications (E&W)
From: HMSO Book Source: OPCS

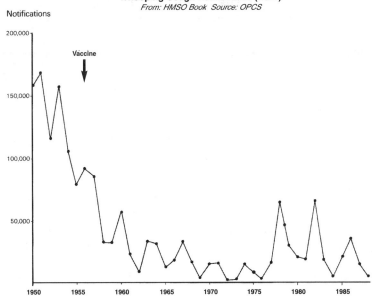

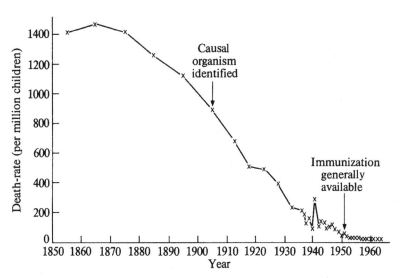

FIGURE 8.12. Whooping cough: death rates of children under 15: England and Wales.

Tetanus notification to ONS
England and Wales (1969-1995)

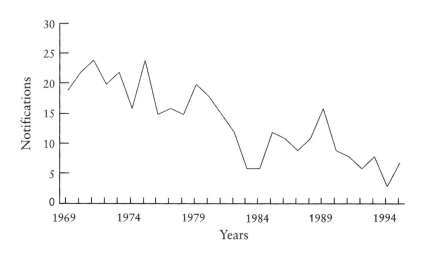

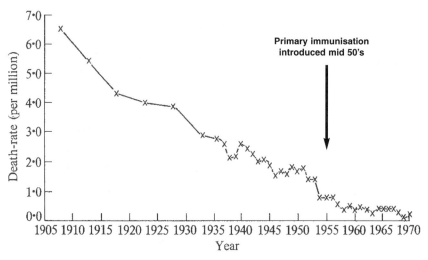

FIGURE 8.11. Tetanus: mean annual death rates: England and Wales.

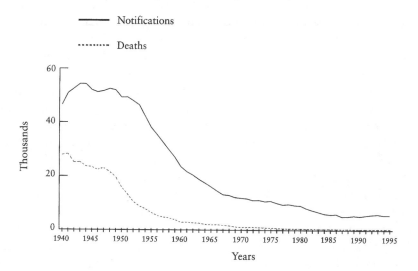

Notifications of tuberculosis and deaths to ONS
England and Wales (1940-1995)

——— Notifications

·········· Deaths

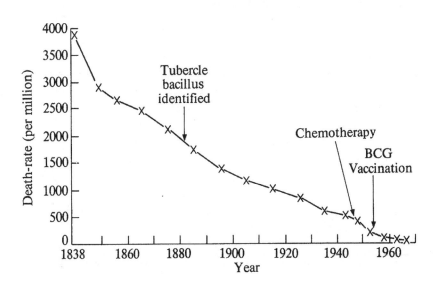

Respiratory tuberculosis: mean annual death-rates E&W.

Tubercle
bacillus
identified

Chemotherapy

BCG
Vaccination

These graphs all highlight that the death rates for these various infections declined dramatically BEFORE vaccines were introduced. It is important to note that the statistics for these graphs are from the SAME government offices that collate the statistics for the graphs in the HMSO book promoting vaccines. They are not collated from studies carried out by people with different vested interests; the same departments that collate the stats for the HMSO book also have the stats for the graphs shown here.

The main factors for these major declines were improvements in health brought about by improved nutrition, less over-crowded living conditions, clean water, sanitation, refrigeration of foods and so on. The healthier the population became then the fewer cases, complications and deaths occurred.

In fact the only illness to have an increased death rate since the 1850's was in fact the first illness to be vaccinated against, smallpox.

In England: Free smallpox vaccines were introduced in 1840 and made compulsory in 1853. Between 1857 and 1859 there were 14,244 deaths from smallpox. After a population rise of 7%, the death rate rose by 40.8% to 20,059 between 1863 and 1865. In 1867 evaders of vaccination were prosecuted. Those left unvaccinated were very few. After a population rise of 9%, the death rate rose by 123% to 44,840, between 1870 and 1872.

The much touted anecdote 'vaccines have eradicated smallpox' cannot be justified by the actual evidence, in fact all of the evidence shows that the smallpox vaccine increased the severity and incidence of smallpox when all other illnesses (that at the time had no vaccines) were on the decline. Where do vaccine promoters get their evidence from, do they in fact have any evidence or is this just a belief?

The belief that falls in vaccine uptake will result in huge outbreaks does not make epidemiological sense. At the beginning of the 1900s scarlet fever accounted for the most deaths amongst the childhood diseases, and yet this disease declined in the same manner as measles, whooping cough, tetanus, diphtheria, TB and so on, such that now it is extremely rare. This was achieved without the introduction of a vaccine; there has never been a vaccine for scarlet fever, it appears that the reduction in scarlet fever deaths and incidence just beat the pharmaceuticals to the post. Had there been a vaccine for scarlet fever, would we still be vaccinating against it now? Promoted by pharmaceuticals, exploiting the fear that it would ravage our children should we fail to vaccinate them.

These graphs clearly show that factors other than vaccines affect health and therefore influence immunity to disease. Otherwise there would always be

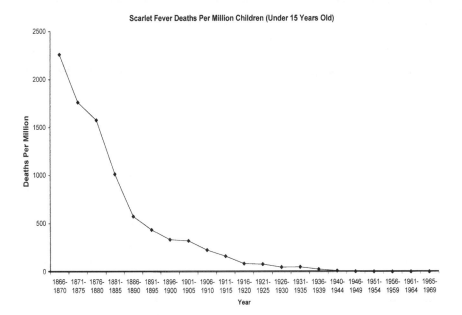

Scarlet Fever Deaths Per Million Children (Under 15 Years Old)

high levels of incidence and mortality with falls occurring only when there was an introduction of a vaccine, and that is clearly not the case.

Often vaccine promoters talk of an unvaccinated child as an unprotected child, this is bad science. You can not 'unprotect' your child by not vaccinating, as that presupposes that the only thing we have protecting us are vaccines, and as the graphs demonstrate, this is not the case. Natural immunity to disease is a natural consequence of general health promotion, you do not need specific vaccine-induced antibodies to be protected against disease, there are billions of microbes that are associated with illnesses that we do not have antibodies to and yet we do not develop the illness.

Incidentally, the word 'epidemic' conjures quite an alarming picture in many people's eyes 'An epidemic is coming', 'there's an epidemic just round the corner'. The idea for most is that if an epidemic hits an area or country that many will succumb to the disease. What is the actual definition of an epidemic? An epidemic is actually quite small: 35 cases in 100,000 population for the case of polio and less for other illnesses. Epidemics affect a very small percentage of the population and therefore not what we have been led to believe through alarming statements from health departments and the media.

STATISTICS, AND MORE STATISTICS.

W e know that there are many factors that affect our health and therefore immunity to disease, but are there any other factors that influence the statistics? What else can make it look like a particular vaccine is working, when in fact it may not?

REPORTING

T he number of cases of disease recorded will not only depend on the actual number of people with those diseases, but just as importantly, will depend on the nature and accuracy of the reporting. There is a tendency to under-report the incidence of a disease in the vaccinated or in a community when vaccine uptake is thought to be high, and similarly over-report the disease in the unvaccinated or when the vaccine uptake is thought to be low.

For example, in the USA a television program, DPT - Vaccine Roulette, shown in April 1982, warned of the dangers of vaccination, especially the whooping cough component (the 'P' part of the DPT vaccine against diphtheria, whooping cough and tetanus) indicating it could cause neurological complications, brain damage and even death. Within months, whooping cough epidemics were reported in the states of Maryland and Wisconsin. It was stated by the Maryland Health Officials that the epidemic was due to parents seeing the documentary and not having their children vaccinated. The cases were analysed by Dr Anthony Morris, an expert on bacterial and viral diseases and a member of the FDA (USA drug regulatory body). In Maryland, 5 of the 41 cases were confirmed; all of them had been vaccinated. In Wisconsin, 16 of the 43 cases were confirmed; all of them had been vaccinated.

Therefore whooping cough cases were being over-reported when the health authorities thought that vaccine uptake was low, and in fact the only confirmed cases were in the vaccinated. A fact that had only come to light because of the investigation, Dr Morris therefore further concluded that whooping cough cases were probably occurring all the time in vaccinated individuals but were not being reported. Therefore illnesses are under-reported in the vaccinated, all of which would create a statistical difference in the numbers of illnesses in the vaccinated compared to the non-vaccinated due to a simple bias in reporting.

So the reliability of reporting is highly questionable. Additionally, the immunisation status is often not highlighted or even established when we are told that vaccine uptake has been responsible for declines in disease or when reductions in uptake are blamed for the outbreaks of disease. For example, in Ireland there are no accurate figures available for the uptake of the MMR from when it was introduced in 1988 until 1997 according to the Irish health department, so they have no way of knowing the effect of the vaccine in that period.

DISEASE CLASSIFICATION

The classification of a disease will have an impact on the number of cases of a disease. For example with polio, prior to 1955 if you had paralytic symptoms arising from a gut microbe, lasting for over 24 hours, this would have been called paralytic poliomyelitis. However, after 1955 the paralysis had to last for anything from 14 to 60 days before it would be classed as paralytic polio. Since the majority of polio cases were resolved within a few days then thousands of cases were reduced to dozens by this simple reclassification. An apparent fall in polio cases at a time that conveniently coincided with the introduction of the polio vaccine.

The system of classifying an illness according to the presence of a micro-organism brings certain problems and inherent inaccuracies. It is possible to have, for instance, a measles-like illness associated with viruses other than the measles virus, and paralytic polio-like illnesses associated with viruses other than polio viruses. We have now distinguished at least two viruses that are associated with symptoms of illness that are exactly the same symptoms as polio: the Coxsackie virus and Echovirus. They are part of a family of viruses of which we have now identified 72, all associated with symptoms that are exactly the same as paralytic poliomyelitis. Therefore, what would previously have been classified as polio will now be classified according to these new viruses. There are also symptoms of polio that look like meningitis and if no bacteria are identified these cases would previously have been added to the numbers of cases of polio, whereas now all such cases are classified as aseptic meningitis. And where no microbe can be identified at all then it will be classified as Guillaine Barre syndrome. So the effects of classification and re-classification of illness dramatically influence the figures, giving an inaccurate epidemiology of the disease.

SYMPTOM SUPPRESSION

Then last but not least the figures relating to the number of cases of an illness do not tell you if the medical procedure of vaccination has actually helped the population or created a deterioration in health. For example, the mumps component of the MMR vaccine in the early 90s was found to be causing mumps meningitis (and was eventually withdrawn). It may have been possible to show reduced cases of mumps but if this was accompanied by increasing cases of meningitis, then it is not possible to see this from a graph that only concerns itself with figures of mumps. This was only discovered after many years of use, so even if the vaccine could reduce the numbers of cases of mumps the important question remains, are we healthier or worse off as a result? Graphs showing declines in incidence of disease do not tell us what is happening to the health of the individual and therefore the whole population.

VACCINATION TRIALS

To identify any problems with a vaccine, proper trials must be conducted and long-term observations carried out. Designing a trial to find out whether a vaccine works, would not be very difficult at all, we would need a control group, i.e. a group of individuals who are not vaccinated to compare with a vaccinated group.

This would need to be a large group and the selection of vaccinated and non-vaccinated would need to be randomized so that statistically you would be comparing groups with an equal variety of healthy, non-healthy, old, young, etc. the trial would also, have to be a 'double-blind' trial, meaning that neither the administrator nor the recipient would be aware of which they were giving or receiving; vaccine or a non-vaccine. This is important because if you have a positive association with being vaccinated it might have an effect on the outcome, it could positively influence your health and this is called the placebo effect. All drugs that are tested on the population have to go through some kind of double-blind, randomised, placebo, controlled trial.

HOW MANY VACCINE TRIALS HAVE BEEN CARRIED OUT IN THIS WAY?

Well, it is extremely rare, since it is said to be unethical. Why unethical? It is said to be unethical to leave one group 'unprotected' to create the placebo group from which to do the comparisons, note that almost all other drugs are required to undergo this procedure. Clearly the supposition is that the advantage of the vaccine must outweigh any disadvantage, the pre-supposition is that the vaccine works, then logically it would be unethical to create a non-vaccinated (placebo) group. This is of course a circular argument, the point of the trial would be to determine that very premise; you cannot know that a vaccine benefit outweighs any disadvantage over and above natural immunity until you carry out a trial.

However one such study was reported in The Lancet, 12 January, 1980, the vaccine studied was the BCG vaccine against TB (tuberculosis). The trial involved 260,000 people comparing an equal sized vaccinated group with a placebo control group. This study was organized after various small studies conducted between 1935 and 1955, produced results that the Lancet states 'varied, strikingly and mysteriously, with protective effects ranging from 0% to 80%.' In fact those 20 years of trials were carried out after a vaccination campaign in a relatively small area of Europe left 72 children dead within a few months of inoculation with the BCG vaccine, a catastrophic event considering the low incidence of the disease and even lower death rate at the time.

The Lancet goes on to state that 'the largest controlled field trial ever done with this vaccine shows not only no evidence of a protective effect but in fact, slightly more tuberculosis cases have appeared in vaccinated than in equal-sized placebo control groups.'

The results of the largest ever field trial carried out on BCG vaccine shows that you were more likely to develop TB had you been vaccinated, than had you not been vaccinated. How did the authorities respond to such a result? We may have expected a re-trial at the very least, or further trials, perhaps a review of vaccine policy for TB and the withdrawal of the vaccine until, at the very least, the development of a better vaccine. However none of the above happened, vaccine policy continued regardless of the results of that trial.

Why was this? Perhaps it could be likened to the opening of Pandora's Box, a medical and political can of worms. Once you start, where would it end? Once you acknowledge the ineffectiveness and side-effects, where do you stop?

Medical professionals are like any other professionals, in that it is very difficult for them to question their core beliefs based on their training, practice and livelihood, even though the evidence suggests that they should. Vaccines are looked upon as one of THE medical wonders of modern medicine and it is often seen as medical heresy to even doubt it.

ILLNESS AND THE IMMUNE SYSTEM

Let's now take a look at our physiology and the basic functioning of the body in a slightly more holistic manner than is common in our everyday medical language. In the diagram we have illustrated a person with the mouth as shown; the mouth leads to a tube which goes into a bag, which is the stomach. The stomach leads into a longer tube, the small intestine. This eventually leads to the large intestine and finally continues out to your anus at the other end.

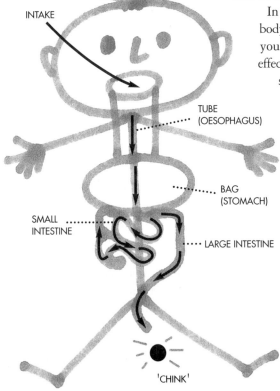

INTAKE

TUBE
(OESOPHAGUS)

BAG
(STOMACH)

SMALL
INTESTINE

LARGE INTESTINE

'CHINK'

In this simplified version of the body, we can imagine that whatever you put in your mouth is effectively still outside of your body, similarly your stomach and intestines are still effectively outside of the body. So for example, if you were to swallow a marble, at some time in the future after your daily evacuation, you would hear a 'chink' - and after the expulsion of that marble at no point did it go inside of your body.

It is only when something pierces your skin that it enters your 'internal spaces' and into your body, your blood, accessing your organs, tissues, and so on. Now about 80% of your immune system actually

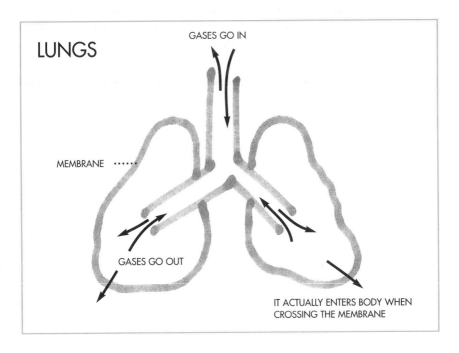

LUNGS

GASES GO IN

MEMBRANE ······

GASES GO OUT

IT ACTUALLY ENTERS BODY WHEN
CROSSING THE MEMBRANE

functions in this 'outside space' of your body. We could do a similar thing with your lungs; one tube leading to two tubes, ending in the convoluted membranes forming the membrane of the lungs. Gases pass in and out, and it is only the ones that go across the membrane that actually enter into your body.

Toxins accumulated in the body are eliminated through the skin, the lungs, the kidneys and the large intestine. The way into the kidneys from your internal body and blood supply are through tubes, one side of the tube is your blood and the other side of the tube is a space. This space is connected to your ureter from both your right and left kidney which is connected to a bag, your bladder, then into one tube your urethra and through that you urinate - therefore once it goes into that space it is now outside of the body. Although we know these spaces are in intimate contact with the body and that substances can be absorbed into the body from here, the point is to create a perspective of how the body functions in eliminating out into these spaces and how important these functions are in immune function and in maintaining health.

So the body has the permanent job of keeping things out that it does not want, and eliminating waste that is naturally produced internally that it similarly doesn't want. That is a large part of our immune function and the main structure involved would be the skin or mucous membrane. Now there are many components associated with those parts of the body:

- White blood cells that can enter any part of that system. They have access to your lymphatic vessels and glands such as tonsils and adenoids
- Non-specific antibodies
- Bacteria that help immune function (there are more micro-organisms in your body than there are your own cells)
- Hairs that filter
- Enzymes able to break down components
- Immune chemicals that coordinate and carry out immune function
- Mucus fluid that can be acidic or the opposite alkaline
- The membrane itself functions as the most important barrier

So when there is a toxic problem and/or an abundance of non-beneficial microbes, these elements operate at the site of toxicity breaking down and digesting unwanted elements so that they can be eliminated from the system.

Now a child's system, from birth, is immature and in the process of developing. The stomach membrane is more porous (leaky) than the adult membrane, therefore allowing things into the blood far more readily than in an adult. Therefore a baby will be initially fed baby milk, ideally breast milk, which has small nutritional components that do not need much breakdown and digesting, these elements are beneficial and will be absorbed very easily across the membrane and therefore into the body of the child. What would happen if you gave your baby meat and two veg from day one? This would poison the child, due to the inability of the child to digest the food, from not having the necessary enzymes to break down the much larger components of food molecules, and a membrane that is unable to keep out all of these elements from the blood, effectively resulting in toxins entering the blood.

THE DIFFERENCE BETWEEN THE REACTION AND THE PROBLEM

So how would the child react to ingesting a potential poison? Initially babies react typically through vomiting and diarrhoea, they don't initially even have the capacity to create a fever, it may take days or even weeks for some babies to develop the capacity to have an inflammatory response. The 'reaction', vomiting and diarrhoea, is therefore a necessary part of the resolution of the problem of toxicity in the gut. Therefore the 'problem' is the toxin accumulation in the digestive tract and the 'reaction' vomiting and diarrhoea, is part of the cure. However, often the current orthodoxy perceives the vomiting and diarrhoea as being the problem itself, rather than being indicative of a problem, so often the problem and reaction are treated as one. In fact generally the real problems are ignored and the reaction itself is seen as the dangerous thing to be stopped. Consequently medication is taken to suppress reactions in an attempt to treat the condition, i.e. drugs to stop diarrhoea and vomiting.

Logically, suppressing the very reaction needed to resolve the problem will make it more likely that the problem remains i.e. in the case of toxic build up in the digestive tract, those poisons will remain in the digestive tract, which will lead to either a recurrence of the reaction (vomiting and diarrhoea) or the body will step-up it's attempt to resolve the situation.

The next step would take the form of an inflammatory response, if the child is able to do this. An inflammatory response is the mechanism whereby the body mobilizes white blood cells to an area of toxicity or dead/injured tissue. To do this, the blood vessels widen in that area, dilation. Secondly the membranes separating the blood from the toxic space (in this instance the gut membrane) and the blood vessel walls themselves become more permeable (leaky), allowing the white blood cells to squeeze out of vessels into the relevant space of the body, leading to symptoms of redness, swelling, pain and heat. The white blood cells once in the appropriate place will break down/digest toxins and dead tissues, preparing them for elimination; again via the process of vomiting and/or diarrhoea.

The aim of the body's response is to keep the toxins out of the bloodstream. So your child's body will mount an inflammatory response at the appropriate site, maybe as a gastritis, laryngitis, sinusitis, cystitis, and so on, to keep the toxins outside the body. Again it is possible from an orthodox medical perspective to perceive the inflammation as the problem itself, giving

INFLAMMATION REACTION CAUSED BY EXCESS TOXINS IN THE DIGESTIVE TRACT

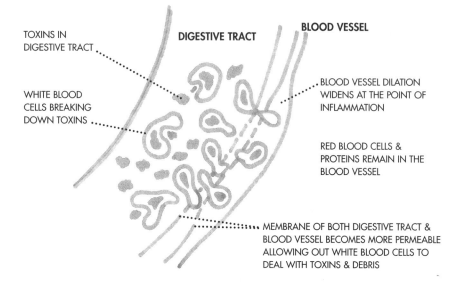

TOXINS IN
DIGESTIVE TRACT

DIGESTIVE TRACT

BLOOD VESSEL

WHITE BLOOD
CELLS BREAKING
DOWN TOXINS

BLOOD VESSEL DILATION
WIDENS AT THE POINT OF
INFLAMMATION

RED BLOOD CELLS &
PROTEINS REMAIN IN THE
BLOOD VESSEL

MEMBRANE OF BOTH DIGESTIVE TRACT &
BLOOD VESSEL BECOMES MORE PERMEABLE
ALLOWING OUT WHITE BLOOD CELLS TO
DEAL WITH TOXINS & DEBRIS

anti-inflammatories to suppress these reactions.

Consequently if toxins are not eliminated from these external spaces, (external from our previous definition including the respiratory, digestive, and urinary tracts) what then happens to them?

In intimate contact with the membranes and without elimination, they have the potential to pass across the membrane and get into the blood, it is also likely that toxins that naturally accumulate in the blood as a result of our normal metabolism build-up within our internal blood system; this then leads to a very different reaction in an attempt to cleanse the body once again. Here we see the mobilization of other white blood cells, in the blood itself; T-cells, B-cells, Natural Killer cells and in some instances the production of antibodies, produced by the B-cells.

You could have a T-cell reaction, which tends to deal with the cells that have been affected by the toxins. If the T-cells fail to deal with the problem, for example, if toxins remain in the blood, then antibody production is called for. Antibodies appear to be the last line of defence for your blood system, and may not be required if the body's cellular immune response is successful, and the required elimination takes place. Antibodies themselves do not destroy anything or eliminate anything, they act as flags indicating where potential problems remain, attracting other elements of the immune system to do their work.

Normally when the toxins are eliminated from the blood they will be eliminated through the skin and/or mucous membranes resulting in rashes. Rash diseases, such as measles, rubella and chickenpox, etc are good examples of what even orthodox medicine calls viral shedding. The importance of this skin elimination of toxins has been demonstrated in an orthodox medical study carried out in Denmark and reported in The Lancet, 5 Jan. 1985. The initial research looked at a group of adults who had measles-specific antibodies present, this meant that they had been in contact with the measles virus but this was not a statement as to whether they were immune or not. Comparing those cases which had produced a typical rash with cases where no rash manifested, the evidence showed that the absence of rash increased the incidence of skin diseases, degenerative diseases of bone and cartilage and certain tumors in adulthood. It was therefore deduced even from an orthodox perspective that the rash, the elimination process, the viral shedding, is an important part of the resolution of illness and should not be suppressed.

VIRAL ILLNESSES

Since the discovery of microbes such as bacteria we have seen similar diseases that are not associated with bacteria. Consequently there are whole classes of illnesses that are thought to be caused by smaller microbes called viruses. However, contrary to the public portrayal of illnesses, the idea that viruses are actually the cause of illness is still a very inadequate theory.

Standard immunology books will state that we are still uncertain as to how the immune system deals with viruses.

There is more evidence to suggest that viruses are broken down elements of cells and therefore part of the clean-up process; because we know that viruses are caused by poisoning cells with various toxins. So it is possible to create viruses within you, by poisoning your cells.

Also we have never been able to prove that viruses cause illness even with our modern technology able to detect viral particles; such infecting viruses (infectosomes) have never been demonstrated in diseased tissue.

It's rather like flies around cow dung, they're always there but they don't actually produce the stuff - thankfully.

So far we have looked at immune responses as 'processes' and therefore it is important to realize that 'immunity' is not a 'thing', it is the result of a system going through a process, and if the immune response is to be more able to cope with conditions after that process, with enhanced immunity, then the system has to 'learn'.

Thinking of the immune system as the possession of chemicals such as antibodies would be like saying education is about having books, but giving your child lots of books does not make them educated. The process of learning to read must take place first. Immunity is not a set of things like a bunch of antibodies, things that you would like to give to an individual; it is a learning process that the body goes through, which results in the person becoming immune i.e. less susceptible to illness.

We are now able to understand that the immune system learns as do many other systems in the human body. This learning process educates and primes the body for future events. It is the same when your child is learning to walk. When ready to learn to walk the initial phase involves standing up, they do inevitably fall down. Much as we would like to teach our children without them falling, we inherently know that this is not possible; learning takes place by a process of trial and error. We therefore minimize the consequences of error, (soft carpet, no dangerous items to fall on etc), however, we cannot eliminate the possibility of error and therefore we reduce the consequences but not the risk of actual error. So after the fall, first the child learns to get up again, the consequences of error, the fall has not been so damaging that the child is unable to try again, so the error of falling is resolved and the child stands again. At some point however we expect the child to learn to balance and that is the point of learning. After learning the child is now less susceptible to falling. If the child had learnt to walk and fallen such that they were seriously injured and shocked, that would have made them less able to get up after and in fact more susceptible to falling.

Likewise when the body eliminates toxins, if there was no learning then the body would be just as susceptible to that toxic build up in the blood system as it was before, like a child that never learns to walk always standing and falling, the body would forever be having rashes and measles. However with real immune learning not only do immune cells learn but the most important elements of the immune system i.e. the membranes also learn. They learn to keep things out that it previously could not i.e. the integrity of the membrane gets stronger, it becomes less penetrable. So you often find that once you have had certain illnesses you are much less likely to suffer from them again and additionally many aspects of the immune system will have been strengthened. This learning is what we call immunity, but it is not rigidly specific, as we initially believed when we thought that specific antibodies were necessary for immunity. However the non-specific nature of immunity is in fact just like any learning, once your child has learnt to walk in one room they could do it in another, or learnt to cross the road they can cross another i.e. there is some specificity but also considerable overlap in our learning capacity.

If that was not the case then we would have to have every single illness possible to become immune to all of those illnesses, and that doesn't happen and is not necessary. Here it is often asked, why did indigenous people succumb so readily to illnesses of their invaders, for example, with the South American Indians with the landing of the Europeans? Here we need to be aware of the distortion of events to suit a prevailing theory. When Europeans landed in South America there were many atrocities carried out to the local people, violence, killing, rape, destruction of homes, stealing resources, enslavement, lifestyle, dietary changes imposed, to name but a few. If we study disease we see they are caused by certain conditions, as would be expected in the above example. Where there are visitors from developed countries to cultures that are subsequently exposed to our so-called viruses we see there is no increased susceptibility to disease, if we really are visitors performing acts that are no more detrimental to our hosts than breathing on them and sharing air-borne microbes, then no disease is created.

CHRONIC DISEASE = PERSISTENT RESPONSE

It is important to realize also that unresolved issues lead us to become more susceptible to our problems. If we look at an emotional example, let's imagine a child on their first day away from their parents, at school. The trauma is 'separation', the reaction is to 'cry', if the expression of their grief, crying, was suppressed i.e. they were told not to cry, made to feel afraid to cry, then the very reaction that helps them to resolve the situation has been suppressed. The problem has of course not been resolved, in fact the problem stays within, and the child becomes sad. Here we demonstrate that if the acute reaction is unsuccessful, it leads to a chronic reaction, the acute is intense and short-lived, the chronic is less intense and long-lived. Whilst in that state of sadness, unresolved grief, the child is in fact more susceptible to separation trauma. Even within their home with their parents they may even get upset when being left alone in a room as a result of this unresolved issue. Unresolved issues lead therefore to chronic weakness.

To continue our story of immune function, if the elimination of blood toxins is unsuccessful then we will observe the build-up of toxins in internal parts of the body, joints, fat, kidneys, liver, and heart valves. This may then lead to inflammatory conditions in those areas, but it may also lead to chronic reactions, vomiting and diarrhoea lead to chronic digestive disturbances; an acute rash could become a chronic rash, (eczema); an acute cough becomes a chronic respiratory illness (asthma).

If we look a little closer at our generalised inflammatory response to blood toxins, we see that during the inflammatory process it is important to get your white blood cells to the appropriate areas and eliminate blood toxicity out beyond the mucous membranes and skin. To accomplish this the membrane becomes more permeable, (more leaky), however this is part of the 'acute reaction' and when the situation is resolved we would expect the membranes to return to the original state and if there has been a positive learning, then the membranes do in fact become stronger as a result of the process.

NOW WHAT HAPPENS WHEN YOU VACCINATE?

Basically you introduce a foreign cocktail into your blood and leave it there. The idea is to produce antibodies as the possession of antibodies was thought to be immunity, but this is an old (pre-1940) idea of immunity. Remember the possession of antibodies no more constitutes immunity than the possession of books constitutes education, if the toxins are not eliminated the process is in fact unresolved and there is no immune learning. Worse still, if the person does react with fever etc i.e. an attempt to mobilize white blood cells with a generalized inflammatory response, then the fever is routinely suppressed with antipyretics and anti-inflammatories such as calpol, paracetomol etc. This is in fact illogical and dangerous, on the one hand you want to stimulate an immune reaction by injecting poisons into the body and at the same time you are asked to suppress the immune reactions. If this does lead to unresolved immune responses we may expect to increase susceptibility to illness not decrease it as with immune learning. One of the ways of demonstrating this, from a physiological point of view, would be to study what happens to the membranes.

It has been demonstrated and reported in medical literature that after vaccination you can get certain blood chemicals that persist in the body long-term, chemicals that should only be there in acute disease. Therefore we are seeing a chronic reaction, and in addition the membranes have been shown to be persistently porous. We are therefore observing the creation of chronic disease reactions in response to vaccination because clearly the body finds it extremely difficult to eliminate poisons that have not entered the body in the manner that we have evolved to react to, and secondly any attempt to actually resolve this is usually suppressed.

SO WHAT IS THE SIGNIFICANCE OF LEAKY MEMBRANES?

You become more susceptible to substances getting into your body, foods, elements in the air we breathe and toxins gaining access to your blood and internal systems. You become sensitised to something if you cannot deal with it. As such allergic reactions are in fact not over-reactions but damage limitation exercises. For example, if a child is exposed to an acute trauma, such as a strong act of violence. The child is unable to accommodate this in their psyche, they cannot deal with the levels of fear it creates, however the effects of the trauma will remain there until it can be resolved at a later date and they will become sensitive to any violence or anything that looks like violence. So if they saw somebody approaching that could appear to be menacing they may over react - that is what we mean by sensitised.

When a vaccine is introduced into the blood, the system becomes more porous and sensitised to those elements within the vaccine. Vaccines contain many elements - foreign proteins, antibiotics, metals, additives and preservatives, which have the potential to cause various sensitivities in some individuals. When a person develops an allergy, this allergy is the result of something that has been given access to the blood. If you are allergic to egg protein this means that egg protein is getting into your blood and you cannot get it out - you are sensitised to egg protein. Usually you find that people with allergies are sensitive to many things, as it is rare to have an allergy to just one thing. The body then produces an antibody and places it on the part of the body that will meet the substance first, i.e. the skin, mouth, nose etc, the body is then instructed to react strongly if there is any contact with that substance, so as not to allow intimate contact with lungs, digestive tract etc. The body knows that if that substance has access to the membranes it will get in and cause problems in the blood. For example, 'pollen is not dangerous', we think, so this must be an over-reaction, however pollen is dangerous in the blood. Large protein molecules, especially from foods, are in fact dangerous in their whole unbroken down state in the blood. We then take antihistamine to stop that reaction and once again the drug suppresses our highly evolved damage-limitation reaction, what we call an allergy, and we allow more of the problem into the blood to affect the internal systems of the body.

In looking at the vaccine process with relation to viruses especially, it is interesting to note, that if we were to inject somebody with just virus, killed or live, what do you think would happen?

Actually nothing; viruses injected into the body are not a natural phenomena, it may be that the body simply doesn't recognise what is occurring. Similarly viruses themselves are not causes but results of disease, so once again the body does not see this as a threat, especially again if the virus has been changed in some way. Therefore to actually get the body to respond to the vaccine, a poison is put in the vaccine specifically to kick the immune system into reacting, this poison is called an adjuvant. Aluminium phosphate or aluminium hydroxide is usually used in the early baby vaccines for this purpose, to get the body to react. This has more potential problems associated with it than possibly mercury, which for a long time was denied as causing problems, and was eventually reduced from some vaccines for the very reasons that were originally denied.

Another inherent problem with vaccine production is the cultivation of virus. This mostly involves growing the virus on animal tissue. Polio virus, for example, is grown on monkey kidney cells and one of the problems with cultivating viruses is that as the specific virus grows, other things will grow too. This creates the issue of contamination; it is actually not physically possible to produce a pure virus, therefore all viral vaccines have a level of contamination that is allowable. The amount of contaminant virus numbers into millions, and some of these artificial contaminants do create problems in humans that may not be apparent in the animal tissue that it has been cultivated on. For example, the polio vaccine has been known to be contaminated with a cancer-causing monkey virus called SV40, since the 1950s, the contamination was allegedly rectified but debate as to liability still continues to this day.

Vaccine virus also needs to be weakened or killed using physical or chemical procedures; the vaccine also contains preservatives, antibiotics, stabilisers, and elements of the genetics of the tissue that the virus was cultured on. This results in a cocktail of components that have the potential to cause a wide range of health problems.

SUSCEPTIBILITY

From a homeopathic view in order to understand illness, including the so-called infectious illness, we need to look at certain issues.

The human being reacts to trauma in order to resolve and where possible to 'learn', the reactions. Therefore the symptoms, are not the problems they are the solution, the trauma is the problem. The traumas are often associated with life-style, poisons in our food and environment, mental and emotional trauma, etc; often we need to address and reduce these to increase health.

We all react in ways that are unique to us and this is called our susceptibility, issues that are not resolved remain and influence our susceptibility, they are also passed on to future generations.

Microbes often aid in the breakdown of diseased tissue and many are the result of disease not the cause. Microbes do not cause serious illness by virtue of the microbe, they are only associated with serious illness if we are seriously ill. Serious illness comes from unresolved issues, which are ultimately caused by severe or persistent trauma and/or persistent suppression.

Therefore as you raise your level of health you become susceptible to different, less severe types of illness. Whether you're exposed to a virus or not there is no such thing as a dangerous virus, just dangerously ill people. All previous attempts to scare and all previous fears of illnesses have never materialized in the manner predicted by those that promote the idea that the disease is determined by the germ; Sars, Bird flu, HIV, Ebola, all illnesses for which we have no effective treatment to destroy the virus and yet these illnesses did not wipe out large sections of the community but merely stayed within a very small section of susceptible people.

From the orthodox medical view we are taught to be afraid of all illness, that immunity can only be obtained by having the illness, that some are too dangerous to have, and if we are exposed to a particular germ we can contract it. Consequently we are being vaccinated for an ever-growing number of diseases, and by the very nature of this theory the number of vaccines recommended will continue to increase. There has been a 700% increase in vaccines over the last 50 years. The medical profession as directed by the pharmaceutical industry presupposes that we require specific antibodies to every disease in order to be protected, and as discussed earlier, antibodies only play a small role in immunity and their presence does not mean that you are protected.

CONSEQUENCES OF ACUTE ILLNESS

The Homeopathic View

There are certain consequences to having acute diseases, (an acute illness being a reaction to an imposed trauma), two of which we have already discussed; resolution leading to learning and unresolved leading to chronic disease. However we can distinguish four main outcomes as follows:

1. The trauma is resolved and you have learnt from the process, your health improves to a higher level than before, therefore less susceptible to the trauma.

2. You resolve the acute but carry on as before, just as susceptible.

3. The problem is not resolved and your health deteriorates to a lower level than before the acute, therefore more susceptible (sensitised).

4. The problem is not resolved resulting in death.

From observing patterns of illness homeopaths have also observed that these unresolved patterns are acquired in one generation and passed on to the next generation. This is called the acquired or inherited miasm in homeopathy. Therefore as the parent develops or not, the later children may be healthier or less healthy than their older siblings.

In homeopathy we find that the children who express their acute illness become healthier and less susceptible to other illnesses, allergies, asthma, and so on. Whereas those who have their acute disease suppressed are more likely to deteriorate and become more susceptible to other conditions. I would like to stress that this is not just a nice coherent theory it is an observation of symptom patterns over at least 200 hundred years of homeopathic cases from many thousands of practitioners.

Homeopaths are trained to watch for all symptoms, making notes of our observations, in order to understand a child's health we have to look at the parents and grandparents' health, which is why your practitioner will ask about the family medical history. This enables the practitioner to understand the child's level of health and potential patterns of illness. We may inherit more from one parent than the other but can only start with a level of health as great as the healthiest of one of our parents.

As each generation's health declines the miasmatic inheritance will also change. These days you will find children developing cancers at a very early age, whereas before it took eighty or ninety years to develop such chronic disease. The children of today are starting at lower levels of health due to the unresolved issues of the parents. The expression of illness, the elimination of toxins and immune learning is what we try to support as holistic practitioners. The aim is to get the body functioning to allow the elimination of stored toxins from the body and to allow the resolution of stored trauma.

Regarding the resolution of so-called infectious disease, a homeopath will be looking for toxin elimination. Generally there are three components to what we are told is an infection:

1. The development of the immune system i.e. the ability of the body to eliminate.
2. The amount and whereabouts of toxicity in the system.
3. The amount of chronic baggage, i.e. unresolved issues carried by the individual.

An acute infectious illness is a crisis of toxicity, that may come about under times of stress; emotional and/or physical. If resolved it may also enable immune learning, which will help to resolve unresolved patterns that have been inherited, and those that have been acquired; illnesses will therefore express differently in different individuals. The same potential illness, associated (not caused) by the same pathogen will be expressed differently because we are individuals with varying degrees of health. Polio virus is associated with a whole host of symptoms from very few, to digestive complaints, to spasm, to paralysis, to brain disorder, to death, the virus is exactly the same in all cases the difference is the patient.

If the elimination process is SUPPRESSED then toxins can move to deeper levels within the body causing more serious consequences. This also results in your ability to eliminate, to be compromised and thus general health moves to a lower level than what you had before the acute. Suppressing continuously diminishes your health, and if the body is unable to have an acute this will lead to what we call chronic disease. Ultimately toxins will affect the nervous system, either chronically as with ADHD, Autism, ME, or acutely with meningitis, encephalitis, poliomyelitis etc.

POLIO

The Polio story is a very good example of the issues surrounding microbes, infectious illness and vaccines.

Polio cases did not follow the usual trend as with other diseases such as, measles, whooping cough and diphtheria. Polio epidemics of the 1950s were occurring in the developed countries - USA and Britain. There were a number of factors that appear to have contributed to the rise in cases at that time:

1. Exposure to DDT poisoning

2. Routine tonsillectomies

3. Removal of appendix

4. History of antibiotics

5. High exposure to sugar

6. Other vaccines given can provoke a case of polio in the recipient

Polio virus, which supposedly causes paralytic poliomyelitis, is actually in all of us. Polio used to be called infantile paralysis or acute flaccid paralysis. The disease is distinctly caused by neurological poisoning as determined by orthodox research in the 40s, 50s and 60s, poisoning due to the advent of insecticides DDT and DDE. It was also noted as early as the 1900s after the use of lead arsenate in the dairy industry. Note that this was not an alternative view at the time and in fact it was renowned to be NOT an infectious disease but a neurological poisoning.

As the insecticides were banned the illnesses diminished, where they continue to be used in developing countries to this day, the illness persists. As discovered they are more severe in children with compromised immune systems i.e. children with: tonsils and/or appendix removed (the tonsils and appendix are a necessary part of our lymphatic system, not an unnecessary tissue as once believed); with a history of antibiotic use (antibiotics upset the important micro-organism balance within the body); exposure to lots of refined sugar affects the blood metabolism, liver and pancreas making us more susceptible to blood toxicity problems; the administration of other vaccines is an immune shock that adds to the levels of toxins the body has to deal with. All of which understandably pre-disposes children to invasive toxicity.

During this time however, there were other research scientists determined to find a microbe in the cases of acute flaccid paralysis and infantile paralysis, so that ultimately they could produce a vaccine. From the poisoned tissue of victims, amongst all manner of debris and toxins, they found polio viruses and this has always been promoted as the cause of the illness though never proved as the cause, consequently the polio vaccine was produced in its various forms to counter the illness. The vaccine has never been responsible for diminishing cases of neurological poisoning which is the true nature of what we now call polio. The illness was hijacked by vaccine producers and its efficacy has never been demonstrated, the virus has never been demonstrated to cause the tissue to become diseased in the natural illness, no infectosomes have ever been found.

There have been two types of polio vaccine, oral and injectable and producers from both sides have accused the other of causing more polio than preventing. In fact polio vaccines, along with all other vaccines, add to the immune load predisposing individuals to more severe illness such as the neurological poisoning now called paralytic poliomyelitis.

The question of swimming pools often arises, is it possible to contract polio from a pool? In theory you can get any gut microbe from a pool, but you would have to ingest the excrement of another individual to be affected by it. Then of course the microbe would be the last of your worries, there are plenty of toxins in human excrement that would create a problem, and your reaction would not be paralytic poliomyelitis. In fact polio has never been contracted from any pool in the UK, and if microbes were to survive in a pool, then it would be poorly maintained and many other reactions would occur before anything resembling paralytic poliomyelitis.

It has been reported that individuals in a household have contracted polio from a child recently taking an oral polio vaccine through contamination of the child's excrement. However this highlights the toxic nature of the oral vaccine, the symptoms of the individual are polio-like but do not lead to long term neurological consequences, this could only happen if the individual is immune-compromised and has their symptoms acutely suppressed. In any event any household that regularly ingests their child's excrement has a hygiene issue (toxins) and are susceptible to illness, believe it or not.

The questions surrounding polio highlight our difficulties in letting go of the old medical paradigm. We all have viruses; polio and millions of others, viruses are the result of disease not the cause, and similarly bacteria are the result of the disease not the cause. Vaccines are a nice idea, (100years ago), but they are naive, they do not create immunity, they sensitise us, are toxic and are dangerous.

TETANUS

Tetanus seems to create a separate issue; the illness is caused by the activity of microbes from a cut and therefore, unlike other illnesses, does appear to be more closely related to vaccination. The tetanus bacteria themselves are widespread and can be found in soil, dust, manure, rust and even in the digestive tract of people. However the issues are the same, firstly the symptoms of tetanus, paralysis and rigidity, are due to poisoning of the nervous system, often the first signs are in the jaw, hence the term lock-jaw. This nerve poisoning is in fact the end result of a disease process that can be avoided once we are clear about the causes.

If a wound contains enough material for bacteria to live on and is covered, with no access to air, then the bacteria will grow without oxygen (anaerobically) this could give rise to the bacterial toxin that could lead to blood poisoning. Therefore shallow cuts and grazes do not pose such a problem and in deeper injuries the first preventative is wound cleaning; this does not require topical antibacterial treatments as the presence of bacteria are not a problem, so long as the debris that they live off are removed. Thus wound cleansing has been recommended in Accident and Emergency departments utilizing tap water only. A drugs and therapeutics bulletin, 25 November 1991, states that antibacterial applications actually slow wound healing making the situation worse, therefore tap water is recommended even in the Accident and Emergency departments of hospitals.

But, if for example, a wound did contain debris, bacteria and no oxygen then the patient would experience blood poisoning, in which case the site would become red and inflamed. Almost all patients in developed countries that are NOT specifically unwell with immune compromised conditions have an immune system and therefore would react successfully to such a wound. In fact tetanus is virtually unheard of in developed countries, vaccines however cannot be used as the reason for this as it is estimated that at least 40% of these populations do not have up-to-date vaccines of tetanus. In the building industry where this figure may be higher and the nature of these wounds are a common everyday occurrence, there is no tetanus. Clearly natural immunity plays a significant role in preventing this illness.

If therefore a deep wound was not cleaned, and there were sufficient bacteria and debris, the wound was covered allowing in no oxygen and the patient was unable to exhibit a successful inflammatory response, then a blood poisoning would develop with concomitant symptoms. This can also be treated, the wound can be surgically cleaned, the bacteria are sensitive to penicillin and there are many alternative treatments for this as well as effective nutritional advice that will help alleviate the problem.

If however this blood poisoning was not dealt with successfully i.e. if in fact the symptoms were suppressed i.e. the inflammation was suppressed then the poison could become invasive and ultimately affect the nervous system. A passive vaccine i.e. tetanus antibodies can be given to help 'marker' the tetanus toxins, but the body will have the job of eliminating this poison from the system, there is also no guarantee that the body will not react to these foreign antibodies increasing the immune load as opposed to helping. In such an instance of an acute problem, when you already have an injury, this passive vaccine of antibodies is not the standard vaccine used in for example the DPT. So there are in fact a whole host of reactions and systems that come into play so that toxins from injuries do not become invasive and affect the nerves, this is actually what the body is designed to do. The risk of this illness is more or less negligible in the developed world, unless the individual is already immune compromised.

But the question still remains; will the vaccine help? Once again we are back to all of the above, the vaccine does not promote a full immune response, associated symptoms i.e. responses are suppressed. Vaccines poison the system directly in the blood and therefore remain in the system adding to the immune burden and possible long-term effects. It has been demonstrated that the immune response to tetanus results in a low T-cell response (high suppressor to helper T-cell activity) and a high B-cell antibody response which may persist. Such a response is similar to the immune compromised response of patients with AIDS, and therefore research on the tetanus vaccine may implicate vaccines as a cause of some immune compromised reactions rather than enhanced immune responses.

As such the tetanus issue runs a parallel to all invasive consequences of any so-called infectious disease. They can all become invasive, whether from the lungs, skin, digestive tract, injuries etc, whatever the point of entry, the issue is the same, if the invasive toxins are not dealt with, then the consequences may eventually affect the nervous system and could lead to the death of the patient, this makes tetanus no different to any other infectious illness you care to look at, measles, mumps, flu, polio, etc.

TRAVEL

So how does this compare to the issue of travel, where we supposedly have not seen these foreign bugs before? Remember the immune system does not work according to whether you have seen the bug before, like learning to cross a different road in a different country you don't have to teach your child the process all over again. So the issue is not the bug, remember again the bugs are the result of disease, the causes of disease are the stresses of our environment and here there are plenty of new conditions that we may have never seen before or may not be well adapted to when we travel.

These conditions may be difficult to adapt to and can therefore lead to symptoms, conditions of hygiene i.e. toxins, different foods, different weather, different stresses, some times more stress, often less stress on holiday. Adrenalin is a natural immune suppressor, work, financial/family anxieties, tea, coffee, cigarettes just a few examples of the conditions to which we respond with adrenalin. There are many adrenalin junkies that are therefore constantly suppressing their immune activity that is what adrenalin does. Go on holiday then the adrenalin diminishes and the immune system starts to repair and eliminate, we then experience symptoms of illness and we see that so many people only fall ill as soon as they start their holiday.

Jet lag, partying, late nights, alcohol, drugs and dehydration, we see symptoms and we suppress with anti-inflammatories, imodium to stop the diarrhoea, pain killers, and headache tablets. If we notice what happens to us, we understand why we respond the way we do, suppression of responses will lead to invasive toxins, we find a bug and we say 'ah ha... that was the cause of my illness'. The microbe was not the cause and a vaccine could not have prevented it. In fact travel vaccines will poison the blood and will predispose you to more illness which is why vaccinated individuals get sicker and why there are no placebo-controlled trials to show the true effects of vaccines.

Yes, but the Ebola virus? Yes, another fantasy, an illness so devastating, caused by a virus capable of killing anyone in its path, at least that's what the public have been led to believe and yet we have no treatment or vaccine for, which raises the question, why hasn't it killed everyone in its path? The source of the virus is unknown; therefore quarantine would only be possible once the patient had symptoms, why is the disease not spreading from whence it came? A quote from the Centre for Disease Control (special pathogens branch) sheds a different light; 'researchers do not understand why some people are able to recover and some do not'.

Once again some people are susceptible and most are not, in fact the illness is prevalent in hospital settings and without further research I do not know what the pre-disposing factors are, but this is an illness like all other illnesses, you cannot travel to an area of virus but an area with certain conditions, you react to the conditions, if reactions are successful no illness is possible, regardless of the presence of virus. If responses are not successful, then increasing health is required, suppression may add to the problem and you need to understand the conditions in order to lighten the load on the patient. Microbes are always there and they change according to the conditions you are subjected to. Severe septicaemia and bacterial proliferation as a result of toxicity may require antibiotics but the illness needs to be addressed or more of the same will result, vaccines play no part in modern health care.

CONCLUSION

For many it takes a while to work with and make use of this health paradigm. Responsibility for our health and our children's health is ours and that does not go away by accepting someone else's word. However, I know that these issues can be easy and knowledge can be used to make the journey easier, like learning to walk; create a safe environment to allow the process and the process will happen, the consequences of failure can be greatly diminished and learning can be enjoyable.

Much of the new research (last 30 years) in immunology corresponds to the principles of holistic medicine. The immune system is a system that 'learns', hence the correlation with the brain and the psyche, consequently the new science of psychoneuroimmunology. As such the immune system learns through small disturbances, as we are subjected to through the food we eat and the air we breathe. We do not need to create crisis, we now know that you can react to immune challenges successfully without ever seeing those substances before, just as a child is able to cross a road and let traffic pass that it has never seen before. Contrary to popular opinion, you can in fact be immune to all kinds of illnesses that you have never had before, through the natural development of the immune system. The specific antibody response only occurs in crisis, one of which has been artificially created by vaccination. Vaccines mimic crisis and then the reactions are suppressed, this is like accepting that your child needs to get run-over by a car in order to learn to cross the road, then trying to mimic that physiologically, just so that they react, then stopping them from reacting. As research scientists are now saying in immunology; crisis is neither necessary nor desirable.

Therefore we are advised to introduce foods gently to children, minimize toxins, if there are errors, reactions will be simple, we do not need projectile vomiting, inflammation and debilitating diarrhoea, but if the toxic load has been such that those reactions do happen, then that was necessary for that child. We will see that resolving illness is our innate ability and is individual, what is good for one person may not be good for another. The ability to react is important and disease is not something out there to fear or to pursue.

When disease conditions are similar then there may be many people with a similar disease, disease reactions arise as they are necessary, remember they are 'reactions' not 'things', if we want to understand disease, understand disease conditions. In a geographical region the population is subjected to similar weather conditions, reactions such as the flu are very closely correlated to changes in weather. Illnesses will sporadically appear at identical times in individuals separated by mountains, rivers and cities and cannot have been transferred by the movement of microbes. In a work environment stresses will appear at similar times, in a family there are similar conditions and similar susceptibilities due to common inheritance.

A child starting nursery will have many colds and green phlegm reactions; we are often told that this is due to bugs being picked up in the nursery. However this does not make microbiological sense, there is no nursery that can contain bugs that are not already in the whole community. More importantly, children at nursery or a similar establishment, especially when this is a new environment, will undergo the stress of separation and the sense of abandonment. From homeopathic case taking we know that this is often accompanied by green snot and clingy behaviour, for which the remedy could be homeopathic pulsatilla. Once the state is resolved the symptoms pass, yet the bugs are still there, as they have always been, and there are no more symptoms. We are able to help the constitution with minute doses of a remedy that is designed to help reactions, not suppress them and we are able to see what the child is reacting to, so that we may be able to reduce their load in order that they learn in a more gentle manner. Part of their load is the trauma of separation from the parents.

However, those that promote the germ paradigm create the sense that disease is out there to get us, the child is exposed to the 'disease' in the nursery, that is where it lurks, other children have it, this mentality preys on fear, it creates more fear, we miss the obvious, and we do not learn the conditions for the disease, so we cannot address them. We feel forced to buy the drug to kill the bug, which resolves nothing, and there has been no immune learning. Worse still, medication may provoke some damage and if we are not aware of the disease conditions we cannot address them.

If one child has a snotty nose or a measles rash then that does not make it important for another child to have one, just as if one child vomits we do not go searching for the vomit bug so we can all be immune. So for many of us the only obstacle is our fear. Therefore I advise you to find practitioners that understand disease, ask questions that reflect your present obstacle, ask until you are satisfied, find systems that do not prey on your fear, and learn to know how to interpret what your body needs. If we learn to listen to ourselves we build trust, if we learn to make connections as to what disturbs us, we create a healthy environment and build compassion for life around us. If we ask the questions we need answers to, we develop from ourselves and we can pass this on to our children. Then the power disseminates from those that exploit our fear to those that would like to empower others - and the whole world can live happily ever after - or at the very least, healthier.

Trevor Gunn, BSc. LCH RSHom, October 2005

USEFUL REFERENCES

1. Comparative graphs; HMSO book, Immunisation against Infectious Disease (1990/96 editions). Incidence of infectious illness from 1950's demonstrating effectiveness of vaccines; Thomas McKeown, The Role of Medicine. Mortality rates from infectious disease from 1850's.

2. Review of BCG vaccine against tuberculosis. Bad news from India; The Lancet Jan 12 1980; 73-74

3. Review in WDDTY, Vol.4 No.6 Dr J Mansfield & Dr D Freed Choking on medicine, effects of bronchodilators in asthmatics

4. JAMA 1994; 272; 592-3 Dr Michel Odent Link between whooping cough vaccine and asthma

5. Ronne T., The Lancet Jan 5 1985; 1-5 Suppression of Measles Rash and the link with chronic disease

6. Natural course of 500 consecutive cases of whooping cough: a general practice population study, Jenkinson D., BMJ Feb 4 1995; 299-302

7. BMJ vol.314 Jun 7 1997; 1692 Paracetamol for fever is unnecessary

8. Drugs & Therapeutics Bulletin volume 29 No.24 25/11/91 Topical antibiotics for wounds do not work

9. 'Facing the world with soul' Robert Sardelle (Lindisfarne Press) Florence Nightingale Quote - no specific diseases, there are specific disease conditions.

10. Evolution & Healing - The Science of Darwinian Medicine Dr.Randolph Nesse, Professor University of Michigan, Dr.George Williams, Professor Emeritus University New York Pub. Phoenix, Orion Books Ltd.

The content of this booklet may be new to many of you, for others it may confirm what you already know. For those of you that need a bit more convincing and for many of us that exist in a plethora of media and drug company paranoia and need a more balanced portrayal of health and illness - subscribe to The Informed Parent, for reading lists, and a regular newsletter, and incidentally, look out for the next book by Trevor Gunn, we shall endeavour to keep you informed!

Magda Taylor, Director of The Informed Parent

Copies of this booklet are available through:
The Informed Parent, P.O Box 4481,
Worthing, West Sussex, BN11 2WH

Tel: 01903 212969

THE *informed* **PARENT**   *www.informedparent.co.uk*

NOTES: